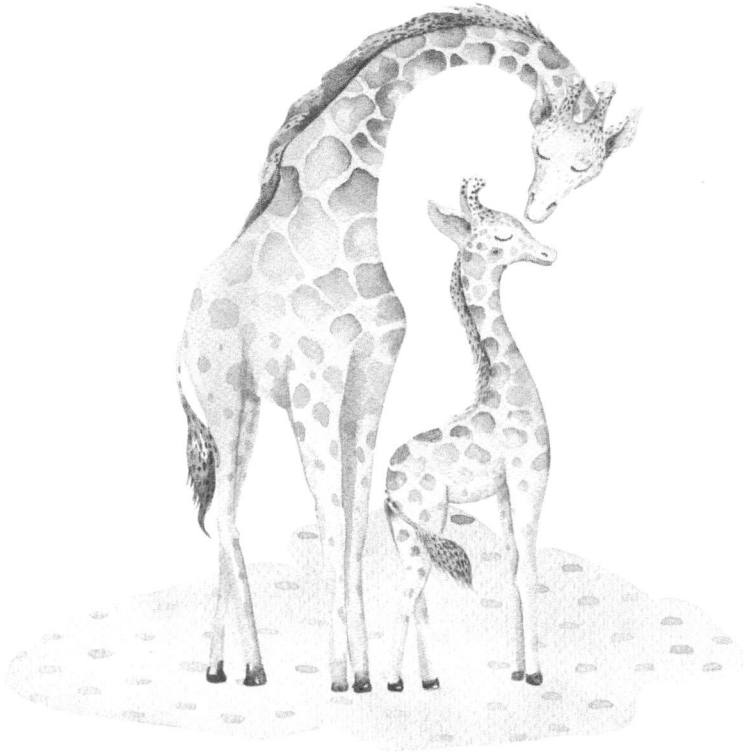

This Pregnancy Journal

BELONGS TO -

_____

_____

_____

_____

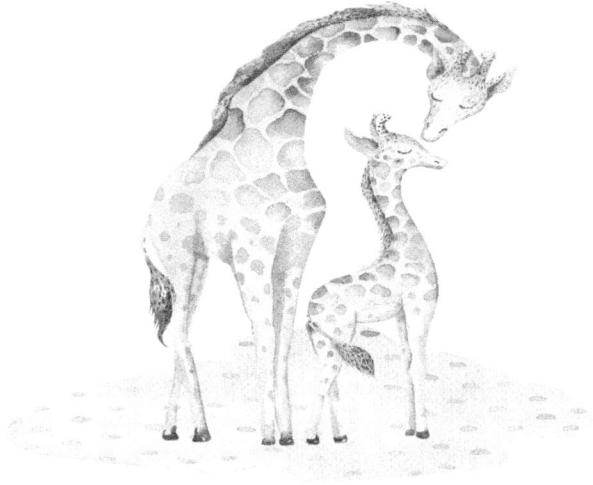

Doctor -

Baby's Due Date -

Date we found out we are expecting -

Date we announced we are expecting -

Heard baby's heart beat for the first time -

Felt baby kick for the first time -

Our baby's nickname -

Pregnancy Cravings -

IMPORTANT CONTACTS

DOCTOR

NAME:

ADDRESS:

EMAIL:

PHONE:

HOSPITAL

NAME:

ADDRESS:

EMAIL:

PHONE:

NAME:

ADDRESS:

EMAIL:

PHONE:

NAME:

ADDRESS:

EMAIL:

PHONE:

NOTES & REMINDERS

IMPORTANT CONTACTS

NAME:

ADDRESS:

✉ EMAIL:

📞 PHONE:

NAME:

ADDRESS:

✉ EMAIL:

📞 PHONE:

NAME:

ADDRESS:

✉ EMAIL:

📞 PHONE:

NAME:

ADDRESS:

✉ EMAIL:

📞 PHONE:

NOTES & REMINDERS

Doctor Appointments

Date	Time	Doctor	Notes

Doctor Appointments

Date	Time	Doctor	Notes

Doctor Appointments

Date	Time	Doctor	Notes

WEEK 1

My Baby's Size

My Weight

Notes

_____

_____

_____

_____

_____

_____

_____

_____

_____

_____

_____

To Do –

☐ _____
☐ _____
☐ _____
☐ _____
☐ _____
☐ _____
☐ _____
☐ _____

WEEK 2

My Baby's Size

My Weight

Notes

_____

_____

_____

_____

_____

_____

_____

_____

_____

_____

_____

To Do –

☐ _____
☐ _____
☐ _____
☐ _____
☐ _____
☐ _____
☐ _____
☐ _____

WEEK 3

My Baby's Size

My Weight

Notes

_____

_____

_____

_____

_____

_____

_____

_____

_____

_____

_____

_____

To Do –

☐ _____
☐ _____
☐ _____
☐ _____
☐ _____
☐ _____
☐ _____
☐ _____

WEEK 4

Notes

_____

_____

_____

_____

_____

_____

_____

_____

_____

_____

_____

To Do –

- ☐ _____
- ☐ _____
- ☐ _____
- ☐ _____
- ☐ _____
- ☐ _____
- ☐ _____
- ☐ _____

WEEK 5

My Baby's Size

My Weight

Notes

_____

_____

_____

_____

_____

_____

_____

_____

_____

_____

_____

To Do –

☐ _____
☐ _____
☐ _____
☐ _____
☐ _____
☐ _____
☐ _____
☐ _____

WEEK 6

Notes

_____

_____

_____

_____

_____

_____

_____

_____

_____

_____

_____

_____

To Do –

☐ _____
☐ _____
☐ _____
☐ _____
☐ _____
☐ _____
☐ _____
☐ _____

WEEK 7

My Baby's Size

My Weight

Notes

_____

_____

_____

_____

_____

_____

_____

_____

_____

_____

_____

_____

To Do –

☐ _____
☐ _____
☐ _____
☐ _____
☐ _____
☐ _____
☐ _____
☐ _____

WEEK 8

My Baby's Size

My Weight

Notes

_____
_____
_____
_____
_____
_____
_____
_____
_____
_____
_____

To Do –

☐ _____
☐ _____
☐ _____
☐ _____
☐ _____
☐ _____
☐ _____
☐ _____

WEEK 9

My Baby's Size

My Weight

Notes

_____

_____

_____

_____

_____

_____

_____

_____

_____

_____

_____

To Do –

☐ _____
☐ _____
☐ _____
☐ _____
☐ _____
☐ _____
☐ _____
☐ _____

WEEK 10

My Baby's Size

My Weight

Notes

_____
_____
_____
_____
_____
_____
_____
_____
_____
_____
_____
_____

To Do –

☐ _____
☐ _____
☐ _____
☐ _____
☐ _____
☐ _____
☐ _____
☐ _____

WEEK 11

Notes

To Do –

WEEK 12

Notes

_____

_____

_____

_____

_____

_____

_____

_____

_____

_____

_____

To Do —

- ☐ _____
- ☐ _____
- ☐ _____
- ☐ _____
- ☐ _____
- ☐ _____
- ☐ _____
- ☐ _____

WEEK 13

Notes

_____
_____
_____
_____
_____
_____
_____
_____
_____
_____
_____

To Do -

☐ _____
☐ _____
☐ _____
☐ _____
☐ _____
☐ _____
☐ _____
☐ _____

WEEK 14

My Baby's Size

My Weight

Notes

_____

_____

_____

_____

_____

_____

_____

_____

_____

_____

_____

To Do –

- [ ] _____
- [ ] _____
- [ ] _____
- [ ] _____
- [ ] _____
- [ ] _____
- [ ] _____
- [ ] _____

WEEK 15

My Baby's Size

My Weight

Notes

_____

_____

_____

_____

_____

_____

_____

_____

_____

_____

_____

_____

_____

To Do –

☐ _____
☐ _____
☐ _____
☐ _____
☐ _____
☐ _____
☐ _____
☐ _____

WEEK 16

My Baby's Size

My Weight

Notes

_____
_____
_____
_____
_____
_____
_____
_____
_____
_____
_____
_____

To Do –

☐ _____
☐ _____
☐ _____
☐ _____
☐ _____
☐ _____
☐ _____
☐ _____

WEEK 17

My Baby's Size

My Weight

Notes

_____

_____

_____

_____

_____

_____

_____

_____

_____

_____

To Do -

- ☐ _____
- ☐ _____
- ☐ _____
- ☐ _____
- ☐ _____
- ☐ _____
- ☐ _____
- ☐ _____

WEEK 18

My Baby's Size

My Weight

Notes

_____

_____

_____

_____

_____

_____

_____

_____

_____

_____

_____

_____

To Do –

☐ _____
☐ _____
☐ _____
☐ _____
☐ _____
☐ _____
☐ _____
☐ _____

WEEK 19

My Baby's Size

My Weight

Notes

_____

_____

_____

_____

_____

_____

_____

_____

_____

_____

_____

_____

To Do –

☐ _____
☐ _____
☐ _____
☐ _____
☐ _____
☐ _____
☐ _____
☐ _____

WEEK 20

My Baby's Size

My Weight

Notes

_____

_____

_____

_____

_____

_____

_____

_____

_____

_____

_____

To Do –

☐ _____
☐ _____
☐ _____
☐ _____
☐ _____
☐ _____
☐ _____
☐ _____

WEEK 21

My Baby's Size

My Weight

Notes

_____
_____
_____
_____
_____
_____
_____
_____
_____
_____
_____

To Do -

- [ ] _____
- [ ] _____
- [ ] _____
- [ ] _____
- [ ] _____
- [ ] _____
- [ ] _____
- [ ] _____

WEEK 22

Notes

_____

_____

_____

_____

_____

_____

_____

_____

_____

_____

_____

To Do –

☐ _____
☐ _____
☐ _____
☐ _____
☐ _____
☐ _____
☐ _____
☐ _____

WEEK 23

My Baby's Size

My Weight

Notes

_____
_____
_____
_____
_____
_____
_____
_____
_____
_____
_____

To Do –

- ☐ _____
- ☐ _____
- ☐ _____
- ☐ _____
- ☐ _____
- ☐ _____
- ☐ _____
- ☐ _____

WEEK 24

My Baby's Size

My Weight

Notes

_____

_____

_____

_____

_____

_____

_____

_____

_____

_____

_____

To Do –

☐ _____

☐ _____

☐ _____

☐ _____

☐ _____

☐ _____

☐ _____

☐ _____

WEEK 25

Notes

To Do –

WEEK 26

My Baby's Size

My Weight

Notes

_____

_____

_____

_____

_____

_____

_____

_____

_____

_____

To Do –

- ☐ _____
- ☐ _____
- ☐ _____
- ☐ _____
- ☐ _____
- ☐ _____
- ☐ _____
- ☐ _____

WEEK 27

My Baby's Size

My Weight

Notes

_____

_____

_____

_____

_____

_____

_____

_____

_____

_____

_____

To Do –

- ☐ _____
- ☐ _____
- ☐ _____
- ☐ _____
- ☐ _____
- ☐ _____
- ☐ _____
- ☐ _____

WEEK 28

My Baby's Size

My Weight

Notes

_____
_____
_____
_____
_____
_____
_____
_____
_____
_____

To Do –

☐ _____
☐ _____
☐ _____
☐ _____
☐ _____
☐ _____
☐ _____
☐ _____

WEEK 29

My Baby's Size

My Weight

Notes

_____
_____
_____
_____
_____
_____
_____
_____
_____
_____
_____

To Do —

☐ _____
☐ _____
☐ _____
☐ _____
☐ _____
☐ _____
☐ _____
☐ _____

WEEK 30

My Baby's Size

My Weight

Notes

_____
_____
_____
_____
_____
_____
_____
_____
_____
_____

To Do –

- ☐ _____
- ☐ _____
- ☐ _____
- ☐ _____
- ☐ _____
- ☐ _____
- ☐ _____
- ☐ _____

WEEK 31

My Baby's Size

My Weight

Notes

_____
_____
_____
_____
_____
_____
_____
_____
_____
_____
_____
_____

To Do –

☐ _____
☐ _____
☐ _____
☐ _____
☐ _____
☐ _____
☐ _____
☐ _____

WEEK 32

My Baby's Size

My Weight

Notes

_____
_____
_____
_____
_____
_____
_____
_____
_____
_____
_____

To Do –

- ☐ _____
- ☐ _____
- ☐ _____
- ☐ _____
- ☐ _____
- ☐ _____
- ☐ _____
- ☐ _____

WEEK 33

Notes

_____

_____

_____

_____

_____

_____

_____

_____

_____

_____

_____

To Do –

☐ _____
☐ _____
☐ _____
☐ _____
☐ _____
☐ _____
☐ _____
☐ _____

WEEK 34

Notes

_____

_____

_____

_____

_____

_____

_____

_____

_____

_____

_____

To Do –

☐ _____
☐ _____
☐ _____
☐ _____
☐ _____
☐ _____
☐ _____
☐ _____

WEEK 35

My Baby's Size

My Weight

Notes

_____

_____

_____

_____

_____

_____

_____

_____

_____

_____

_____

To Do —

- ☐ _____
- ☐ _____
- ☐ _____
- ☐ _____
- ☐ _____
- ☐ _____
- ☐ _____
- ☐ _____

WEEK 36

Notes

_____

_____

_____

_____

_____

_____

_____

_____

_____

_____

_____

To Do –

- ☐ _____
- ☐ _____
- ☐ _____
- ☐ _____
- ☐ _____
- ☐ _____
- ☐ _____
- ☐ _____

WEEK 37

My Baby's Size

My Weight

Notes

_____

_____

_____

_____

_____

_____

_____

_____

_____

_____

_____

To Do –

- [ ] _____
- [ ] _____
- [ ] _____
- [ ] _____
- [ ] _____
- [ ] _____
- [ ] _____
- [ ] _____

WEEK 38

My Baby's Size

My Weight

Notes

_____
_____
_____
_____
_____
_____
_____
_____
_____
_____

To Do –

- ☐ _____
- ☐ _____
- ☐ _____
- ☐ _____
- ☐ _____
- ☐ _____
- ☐ _____
- ☐ _____

WEEK 39

Notes

To Do —

☐
☐
☐
☐
☐
☐
☐
☐

WEEK 40

Notes

_____
_____
_____
_____
_____
_____
_____
_____
_____
_____
_____
_____

To Do –

- ☐ _____
- ☐ _____
- ☐ _____
- ☐ _____
- ☐ _____
- ☐ _____
- ☐ _____
- ☐ _____

WEEK 41

Notes

_____

_____

_____

_____

_____

_____

_____

_____

_____

_____

To Do –

☐ _____
☐ _____
☐ _____
☐ _____
☐ _____
☐ _____
☐ _____
☐ _____

WEEK 42

My Baby's Size

My Weight

Notes

_____

_____

_____

_____

_____

_____

_____

_____

_____

_____

_____

To Do –

☐ _____
☐ _____
☐ _____
☐ _____
☐ _____
☐ _____
☐ _____
☐ _____

Notes

THINGS WE NEED TO BUY

BUB	✓	BUB	✓

THINGS WE NEED TO BUY

NURSERY	✓	NURSERY	✓

Birth Plan

Birth Plan

Hospital Packing List

Hospital Packing List

BABY NAMES - Girls

BABY NAMES - Boys

NURSERY DESIGN IDEAS

NURSERY DESIGN IDEAS

Letter to our Baby

Letter to our Baby

Welcome
TO THE WORLD
Little One

Name -

Date -

Time -

Weight -

Went home -

Visitors

Gifts

_____

_____

_____

_____

_____

_____

_____

_____

_____

_____

_____

Notes

Notes

Notes

Notes

Notes

Notes

Notes

Notes

Notes

Notes

Notes

Notes

Notes

Notes

Notes

Notes

Notes

Notes

Notes

Notes

Notes

Notes

Notes

Notes

Notes

Notes

Notes

Notes

Notes

Notes

Notes

Notes

Notes

Notes

Notes

Notes

Notes

Notes

Notes

Notes

Notes

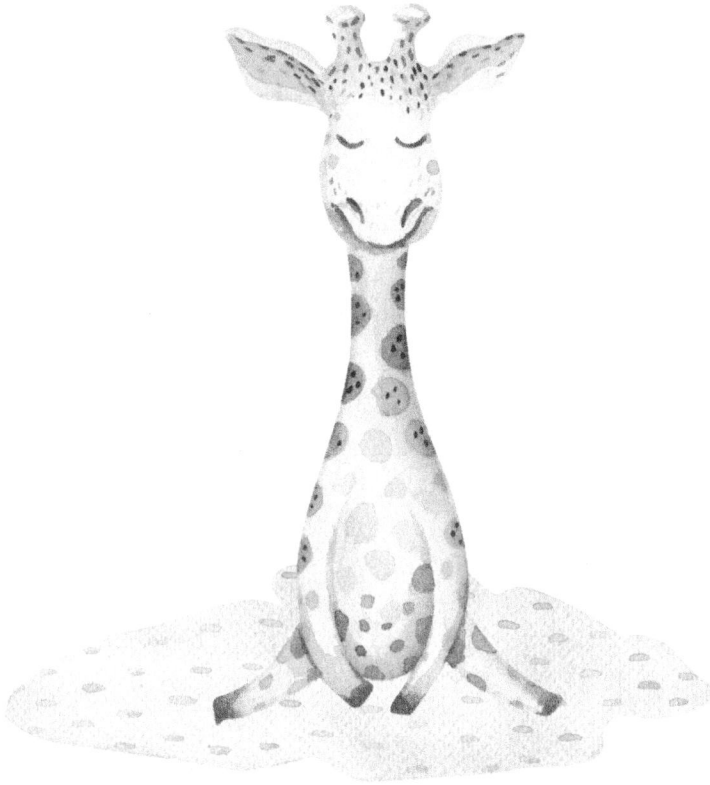

Welcome to the world, little one!